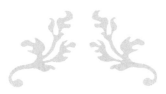

USING SOURSOP FOR CANCER

Using Soursop for Cancer: A Guide to the Treatment of All Types of Cancer Using Graviola Leaves and Fruit Plus 10 Home-made Recipes of Your Favorite Guanabana

Dr. Angie Bairot

Contents

ABOUT

Soursop fruits grow on flowering, evergreen trees native to the tropical regions of Southeast Asia, Africa and South America. The fruit is relatively large in comparison with its small, fast growing plant that reaches up to 10 meters tall. Scientifically known as Annona muricata, soursop fruit is also called by several other names that include graviola, guanabana, custard apple, brazilian paw paw and cherimoya. The heart-shaped fruit with its soft fleshy spines and a rough green skin is an effective cure against dangerous debilitating diseases. In most countries, people make use of the leaves, bark and roots of the tree for traditional remedies.

Soursop fruits have been stated as a medical panacea against variety of illnesses for long. The life-giving properties are due to the following contents.

Vitamin C- A natural antioxidant, it helps in enhancing the immune system and slowing the ageing process.

Phosphorus- This essential mineral aids in bone mass formation and prevents osteoporosis.

Using Soursop for Cancer

Potassium- Highly beneficial in deterring hypertension.

Rich in Fiber- Fibrous content in soursop is highly nutritional and delightful that helps in lowering cholesterol and maintains for bowel regularity.

Iron- A natural source for supplementing our daily iron requirements and preventing anemia.

Rich in vitamin contents B1, B2

Medicinal Aids- Soursop is a healthy and delicious fruit that is used medicinally for treating illnesses ranging from worms to stomach ailments and other lethal diseases.

The seeds contain anti-emetic properties that can be used as a treatment against vomiting.

Its fresh crushed leaves, when applied upon skin eruptions, promote quick healing.

The leaf decoction is quite effective for bedbugs and head lice.

The fruit juice, if taken orally can act as a remedy for hematuria, liver ailments and urethritis.

Using Soursop for Cancer

The juice of the fruit when taken during fasting is believed to cause relief against leprosy and liver ailments.

A decoction of leaves or young shoots is considered a remedy for fever, indigestion, dysentery, diarrhea, coughs, catarrh and gall bladder trouble.

The mashed leaves are often used as poultice for alleviating rheumatism, eczema and some other skin diseases.

The flowers of soursop plant are believed to assuage catarrh.

The prickly long green fruit is an effective cancer remedy that happens to kill malignant cancerous cells up to 10000 times more efficiently than the traditional chemotherapy drugs. Soursop fruit is a broad spectrum antimicrobial agent for both fungal and bacterial infections, is quite effective against worms and parasites, can lower high blood pressure and is often used for stress, depression and nervous disorders. The extracts of this miraculous fruit can

Using Soursop for Cancer

effectively target and kill 12 types of cancer including breast, prostrate, pancreatic, lung and colon cancer.

CANCER

Cancer is a broad term. It describes the disease that results when cellular changes cause the uncontrolled growth and division of cells.

Some types of cancer cause rapid cell growth, while others cause cells to grow and divide at a slower rate.

Certain forms of cancer result in visible growths called tumors, while others, such as leukemia, do not.

Most of the body's cells have specific functions and fixed lifespans. While it may sound like a bad thing, cell death is part of a natural and beneficial phenomenon called apoptosis.

A cell receives instructions to die so that the body can replace it with a newer cell that functions better. Cancerous cells lack the components that instruct them to stop dividing and to die.

As a result, they build up in the body, using oxygen and nutrients that would usually nourish other cells. Cancerous cells can form tumors, impair the immune system and cause other changes that prevent the body from functioning regularly.

Using Soursop for Cancer

Cancerous cells may appear in one area, then spread via the lymph nodes. These are clusters of immune cells located throughout the body.

Causes of Cancer

There are many causes of cancer, and some are preventable.

For example, over 480,000 people die in the U.S. each year from smoking cigarettes, according to data reported in 2014.

In addition to smoking, risk factors for cancer include:

- Heavy alcohol consumption
- Excess body weight
- Physical inactivity
- Poor nutrition

Other causes of cancer are not preventable. Currently, the most significant unpreventable risk factor is age. According to the American Cancer Society, doctors in the U.S. diagnose 87 percent of cancer cases in people ages 50 years or older.

Using Soursop for Cancer

Symptoms of Cancer

Symptoms and signs of cancer depend on the type of cancer, where it is located, and/or where the cancer cells have spread. For example, breast cancer may present as a lump in the breast or as nipple discharge while metastatic breast cancer may present with symptoms of pain (if spread to bones), extreme fatigue (lungs), or seizures (brain). A few patients show no signs or symptoms until the cancer is far advanced.

The American Cancer Society describes seven warning signs and/or symptoms that a cancer may be present, and which should prompt a person to seek medical attention. The word CAUTION can help you remember these.

- Change in bowel or bladder habits
- A sore throat that does not heal
- Unusual bleeding or discharge (for example, nipple secretions or a "sore" that will not heal that oozes material)
- Thickening or lump in the breast, testicles, or elsewhere

Using Soursop for Cancer

- Indigestion (usually chronic) or difficulty swallowing
- Obvious change in the size, color, shape, or thickness of a wart or mole
- Nagging cough or hoarseness

Other signs or symptoms may also alert you or your doctor to the possibility of your having some form of cancer. These include the following:

- Unexplained loss of weight or loss of appetite
- A new type of pain in the bones or other parts of the body that may be steadily worsening, or come and go, but is unlike previous pains one has had before
- Persistent fatigue, nausea, or vomiting
- Unexplained low-grade fevers with may be either persistent or come and go
- Recurring infections which will not clear with usual treatment

Using Soursop for Cancer

Anyone with these signs and symptoms should consult their doctor; these symptoms may also arise from noncancerous conditions.

Many cancers will present with some of the above general symptoms but often have one or more symptoms that are more specific for the cancer type. For example, lung cancer may present with common symptoms of pain, but usually the pain is located in the chest. The patient may have unusual bleeding, but the bleeding usually occurs when the patient coughs. Lung cancer patients often become short of breath and then become very fatigued.

Types of Cancer

There are over 200 types of cancer; far too numerous to include in this book. However, the NCI lists several general categories. This list is expanded below to list more specific types of cancers found in each general category; it is not all inclusive and the cancers listed in quotes are the general names of some cancers:

Carcinoma: Cancer that begins in the skin or in tissues that line or cover internal organs -- "skin, lung, colon, pancreatic, ovarian cancers," epithelial, squamous and basal cell carcinomas, melanomas, papillomas, and adenomas

Sarcoma: Cancer that begins in bone, cartilage, fat, muscle, blood vessels, or other connective or supportive tissue -- "bone, soft tissue cancers," osteosarcoma, synovial sarcoma, liposarcoma, angiosarcoma, rhabdosarcoma, and fibrosarcoma

Leukemia: Cancer that starts in blood-forming tissue such as the bone marrow and causes large numbers of abnormal blood cells to be produced and enter the blood -- "leukemia," lymphoblastic leukemias (ALL and CLL), myelogenous leukemias (AML and CML), T-cell leukemia, and hairy-cell leukemia

Lymphoma and myeloma: Cancers that begin in the cells of the immune system -- "lymphoma," T-cell lymphomas, B-cell lymphomas, Hodgkin lymphomas, non-Hodgkin lymphoma, and lymphoproliferative lymphomas

Central nervous system cancers: Cancers that begin in the tissues of the brain and spinal cord -- "brain and spinal cord tumors," gliomas, meningiomas, pituitary adenomas, vestibular schwannomas, primary CNS lymphomas, and primitive neuroectodermal tumors

Not included in the above types listed are metastatic cancers; this is because metastatic cancer cells usually arise from a cell type listed above and the major difference from the above types is that these cells are now present in a tissue from which the cancer cells did not originally develop. Consequently, if the terms "metastatic cancer" is used, for accuracy, the tissue from which the cancer cells arose should be included. For example, a patient may say they have or are diagnosed with "metastatic cancer" but the more accurate statement is "metastatic (breast, lung, colon, or other type) cancer with spread to the organ in which it has been found." Another example is the following: A doctor describing a man whose prostate cancer has spread to his bones should say the man has metastatic prostate cancer to bone. This is not "bone cancer," which would be cancer that started in the bone cells. Metastatic prostate cancer to bone is treated differently than lung cancer to bone.

Diagnosis of Cancer

Some cancers are diagnosed during routine screening examinations. These are usually tests that are routinely done at a certain age. Many cancers are discovered when you present to your health care professional with specific symptoms.

A physical exam and medical history, especially the history of symptoms, are the first steps in diagnosing cancer. In many instances, the medical caregiver will order a number of tests, most of which will be determined by the type of cancer and where it is suspected to be located in or on the person's body. In addition, most caregivers will order a complete blood count, electrolyte levels and, in some cases, other blood studies that may give additional information.

Imaging studies are commonly used to help physicians detect abnormalities in the body that may be cancer. X-rays, CT and MRI scans, and ultrasound are common tools used to examine the body. Other tests such as endoscopy, which with variations in the equipment used, can allow visualization of tissues in the intestinal tract, throat, and bronchi that may be cancerous. In areas that cannot be well visualized (inside bones or some lymph nodes, for example), radionuclide scanning is often used. The test involves ingestion or IV injection of a weakly radioactive substance that can be concentrated and detected in abnormal tissue.

The preceding tests can be very good at localizing abnormalities in the body; many clinicians consider that some of the tests provide presumptive evidence for the diagnosis of cancer. However, in virtually all patients, the definitive diagnosis of cancer is based on the examination of a tissue sample taken in a procedure called a biopsy from the tissue that may be cancerous, and then analyzed by a pathologist. Some biopsy samples are relatively simple to procure (for example, skin biopsy or intestinal tissue biopsy done with a device called an endoscope equipped with a biopsy attachment). Other biopsies may require as little as a carefully guided needle, or as much as a surgery (for example, brain tissue or lymph node biopsy). In some instances, the surgery to diagnose the cancer may result in a cure if all of the cancerous tissue is removed at the time of biopsy.

The biopsy can provide more than the definitive diagnosis of cancer; it can identify the cancer type (for example, the type of tissue found may indicate that the sample is from a primary [started there] or metastatic type of brain cancer [spread from another primary tumor arising elsewhere in the body]) and thereby help to stage the cancer. The stage, or cancer staging, is a way for clinicians and researchers to estimate how extensive the cancer is in the patient's body.

Is the cancer that has been found localized to its site of origin, or is it spread from that site to other tissues? A localized cancer is said to be at an early stage, while one which has spread is at and advanced stage.

SOURSOP AND ITS HEALTH BENEFIT

Soursop is a common name for the fruit of the Annona muricata tree. The dark green, prickly, heart shaped fruit grows in tropical and subtropical regions of the world.

Some other common names for it include:

- Graviola
- Guanabana
- Guyabano
- Brazilian paw paw
- Custard apple

People describe the flavor of soursop as a combination of strawberry and apple, with hints of citrus. It smells like pineapple and has a creamy texture inside, similar to that of a banana.

People often use the fruit to make beverages, ice-creams, and syrups.

Those in Africa, the Caribbean, and South America use most parts of the plant — including the leaves, fruits, and seeds — in their traditional medicine.

Using Soursop for Cancer

The fruit contains many minerals, including calcium, magnesium, and iron. It also provides 46.4 milligrams (mg) of vitamin C in one cup of pulp, which is over half the recommended daily amount for adults. For context, females need 75 mg of vitamin C per day, and males need 90 mg.

Using Soursop for Cancer

Health Benefits of Soursop

Sour-sop (Graviola) is a fruit of Annona muricata, a broadleaf evergreen tree, native to Mexico, Central and South America. It is an edible fruit, with so many healing powers. The health benefits of soursop juice are numerous because all the parts have medicinal value.

1. Cancer treatment

One of the health benefits of soursop leaves is seen in its ability to prevent cancer and tumours. This is due to the presence of antioxidant substances like acetogenins, alkaloids and quinolones in them. Some research has also been done to get the exact detail of soursop medicinal value.

The study further revealed that the presence of acetogenins in soursop makes it an alternative for cancer treatment. It also stated that soursop is antimicrobial in nature hence an excellent option for treating breast, lungs, prostate and pancreatic cancer.

2. Treatment of Insomnia

The health benefits of soursop juice are seen in its ability to relieve one from stress. It has some anti-inflammatory and relieving power, which makes it an excellent suit for managing anxiety, stress and insomnia or difficulty to sleep.

3. It Control Parasites in the Gut
The antiparasitic nature of soursop has made it a well-known treatment for parasitic infections in most parts of Southern America where parasitic infections are prone. By drinking a tea from the leaves of the tree, you can purify your gastrointestinal system.

4. The Anti-inflammatory Power
The anti-inflammatory property of soursop makes it an excellent suit for managing arthritis. Apply the extracts from soursop on the affected area to easily stop the pain and also hasten the healing process.

5. It Clears Respiratory Problems
The soursop medicinal value helps to clear the airways and relieve congestion in the body. It also helps to clear mucus and phlegm where pathogens may live in the body hence, speeding up the healing process

6. Promote a Healthy Skin
Crushed seeds of soursop have anti ageing power when mixed with your cream. Apply the creams on your skin to prevent premature ageing and other microbial infections.

7. It Boosts the Immune System

The presence of abundant vitamin C in soursop fruits helps to stimulate the production of white blood cells which helps to protect the body. Frequent consumption of soursop juice can help improve the overall health of an individual. The presence of antioxidant substances in it further helps to neutralize free radical substances and its effects.

8. Pain Reliever

According to reports, one of the health benefits of soursop leaves is its ability to relieve pain. Soursop has an analgesic property which helps to relieve pain. Extract the water in the leaves either by quizzing, chewing or any other means and apply the liquid to the affected area at least once in a day until you become better.

9. Enhances Gastrointestinal Health

The soursop medicinal value has been known for decades. Being rich in vitamin C, it has been in use as a natural drug to cure dysentery and scurvy. The soursop juice is also a good diuretic substance which can detoxify the gastrointestinal tract and expel all the toxins and salts from the body. The presence of anti-inflammatory substances in soursop helps to purify the gut.

10. For Diabetes Prevention

The health benefits of soursop leaves for diabetic prevention is of great importance. Some researchers have confirmed that the leaves of soursop can stabilize the blood glucose level in our body at the normal range, between 70 mg up to 120 mg.

Soursop medicinal value is known almost everywhere in the world mostly for its activeness against any sickness that can cause diabetes. Examples of such disease are high blood sugar levels and obesity.

11. It Prevents and Cures Diseases Caused by Uric Acid

Soursop being natural drugs that fight many ailments, can protect you from any sickness related to uric acid, for example, gout. It can also cure the gout infection if you have contracted it. Boil the leaves with water and take it in the morning and evening until you regain your self.

12. Remedy for Boils

A boil is a growth that can occur on any part of the body. In some cases, they transform into infections if not treated properly and damage your skin or face.

Hence, the soursop medicinal value of the leave comes in. In order to get the best result, you get the fresh sour-sop leaves of the plant, squizz it and rub at the affected area until it clears.

13. The Health Benefits of sour-sop leaves in Treating Eczema

One of the health benefits of Sour-sop leaves is its natural remedy for most diseases and it can also cure eczema. This can be achieved by rubbing the extracts from the leaves on the affected area.

14. Treatment of Rheumatism

Rheumatism is bacterial infections that affect the joints and waist of mostly adult people. The health benefits of sour-sop leaves can never be exhausted as it helps to cure the pains caused by arthritis.

Crush some leaves of sour-sop until they become tiny, apply it on the affected area or you soak it in water and drink the liquids till you get better.

15. Sour-sop Useful in Treating Hemorrhoids

A haemorrhoid is a disease that affects the rectum causing the rectum to be bleeding. Sour-sop leaves being antimicrobial, offer protection to your rectum and also halt the rectum from bleeding. It also strengthens the muscles around the rectum and makes them more fit to control haemorrhoid.

SOURSOP FOR CANCER

AGEs derived from the leaf of the plant have shown cytotoxic effects on breast cancer cells in laboratory studies. Researchers have found that purified individual AGEs, and combinations of them, work against breast cancer cells in test tube studies.

Laboratory studies indicate that leaf extracts from the plant are cytotoxic to cells in different types of cancer, including:

- Melanoma
- Skin cancer on the head and neck
- Pancreatic cancer
- Colorectal cancer
- Liver cancer
- Lung cancer

The researchers also showed that extracts from different parts of the plant were cytotoxic to blood cancer cells. The parts of the plant were:

- The leaf
- The pericarp, which is the part of the fruit formed from the ovary

Using Soursop for Cancer

- The seeds
- The stem

Scientists use different solvents to extract the beneficial compounds from the plant, including ethanol, methanol, and chloroform.

Soursop shows antioxidant activity. Antioxidants counteract oxidative stress, which can cause damage and disease in a person's body.

In addition, laboratory research on cancer cells and animal tissue suggests that soursop can:

- Suppress prostate cancer cells and reduce prostate size in rats
- Cause apoptosis (cell death) of lung cancer cells
- Inhibit the migration and invasion of colon cancer cells
- Stabilize breast cancer cells
- Prevent dna damage in the breast tissue of mice

Using Soursop for Cancer

How to Make Soursop Tea
Directions:

- Boil 1 liter of water, then take 15 soursop dry leaves (fresh or dried ones both have same value) and 1 small stem, cut into small pieces and put into the boiling water.
- Don't close the vessel and Continue to boil the water on small flame for 30 mins,until the water evaporates to 500 ml .
- Now the soursop tea is ready to drink. Drink 1 cup (165ml) filtered soursop tea hot or warm or cool , 3 times every day, in the morning, afternoon and in the night.
- For better taste you can add 1/2 spoon of lime juice ,2 pudina leafs and add some honey (not sugar).

After drinking, the body may feel the effects of heat, but no side effects. To cool the body drink 3 glasses of fresh watermelon juice, and drink 3 glasses of goats milk every day. In 2 weeks time you can feel the benefits of soursop yourself, and in 4 weeks time the improvements can be felt clearly.

Using Soursop for Cancer

Note: Drink soursop tea 30 minutes before eating.

Dosing

The appropriate dose of graviola depends on several factors such as the user's age, health, and several other conditions. At this time there is not enough scientific information to determine an appropriate range of doses for graviola.

Be sure to follow relevant directions on product labels and consult your pharmacist or physician or other healthcare professional before using.

Side effects

We don't know much about how graviola affects the body. But some chemicals in graviola concern scientists. It may cause nerve changes and movement disorders.

The nerve changes may cause symptoms like Parkinson's disease. Laboratory research has found that some substances in graviola can cause nerve damage. It crosses into the brain from the bloodstream.

One research study has looked at Caribbeans eating large amounts of graviola. It found that they were more likely to develop certain nerve changes. They were also more likely to have hallucinations.

Studies on animals found that graviola may lower blood sugar and blood pressure. Talk to your doctor first before taking graviola if you have diabetes or high blood pressure. Graviola may also cause damage to your kidneys and liver if taken frequently.

It is unlikely that drinks or foods containing graviola could harm you when taken as part of a normal diet.

Talk to your doctor before taking any kind of complementary or alternative therapy.

BONUS: 10 Favorite Graviola (Sour sop) Fruit Recipes

1. Vegan Soursop Ginger Lime Smoothie
Total Time: 20 Minutes

Ingredients

- 1 soursop (ripe, approximately 1 lb.)
- 3 cups water (filtered, almond or hemp milk)
- 1 teaspoon ginger (grated)
- 1 lime (juiced)
- 1 teaspoon nutmeg
- 1 tablespoon vanilla extract (organic)
- 2 tablespoons stevia (organic, or coconut palm sugar, optional)

Directions

1. Wash the soursop well under running water.
2. Peel the soursop by hand revealing the fleshy fruit inside.
3. Put flesh in a large mixing bowl and remove all the seeds.

4. Put the soursop fruit into your blender. (I use a VitaMix.)

5. Add 1 1/2 to 2 cups of your liquid of choice.

6. Blend on high until the ingredients are pulverized and smooth.

7. Add more liquid, if desired, for a thinner consistency.

8. Add nutmeg, lime juice and vanilla and blend again.

9. Taste and add a little stevia, coconut palm sugar, banana or dried dates, if a sweeter taste is desired. (Optional)

2. Quijada's Soursop Mousse
Total Time: 70 Minutes

Ingredients

- 1 meringue
- 1 tablespoon agar (powder)
- 1 1/2 cups soursop (Pulp, thawed)
- 1/2 cup coconut milk (full –fat)
- 1 cup organic cane sugar
- 1 pinch sea salt
- 3 tablespoons lemon juice
- 1 tablespoon cornstarch (organic, dissolved in 2 tablespoons/ 24g/ 0.85oz of water, room temperature)
- 1 teaspoon agar (powder)
- 1 cup mango (Puree)
- 1 tablespoon lemon juice
- 1 tablespoon organic cane sugar

3. Molea's Soursop Mousse
Total Time: 70 Minutes

Ingredients

- 1 meringue
- 1 tablespoon agar (powder)
- 1 1/2 cups soursop (Pulp, thawed)
- 1/2 cup coconut milk (full –fat)
- 1 cup organic cane sugar
- 1 pinch sea salt
- 3 tablespoons lemon juice
- 1 tablespoon cornstarch (organic, dissolved in 2 tablespoons/ 24g/ 0.85oz of water, room temperature)
- 1 teaspoon agar (powder)
- 1 cup mango (Puree)
- 1 tablespoon lemon juice
- 1 tablespoon organic cane sugar

Directions

Make the Vegan Meringue.

1. In a medium saucepan, pour the soursop puree over the agar; do not stir or heat. Set aside for 10 minutes or longer to allow the agar to hydrate.

2. Whisk the coconut milk, lemon juice, sugar, and salt into the bloomed agar. Bring to a simmer, whisking frequently until sugar has dissolved. Make sure you whisk the bottom and the walls of the pot, coconut milk burns easily.

3. Stir the cornstarch and water with a fork to incorporate the starch. Whisking constantly, add the slurry to the simmering liquid. Bring to a full boil, lower the heat to maintain a low boil, and cook for a minute or so. The mixture will feel thicker almost immediately. Remove the saucepan from the heat.

4. Pour the mixture into a shallow bowl and cool to room temperature. Refrigerate 20 to 30 minutes, or until the gel is very firm. Once firm, cream in a food processor using the S blade, pulse gently until creamy.

5. Transfer the mixture to a mixing bowl and add 1 spoonful of vegan meringue, using a rubber

spatula, incorporate the meringue into the mixture with folding motions. Repeat the previous step slowly, until you add approximately 1 cup of meringue. Keep in mind that if you add too much meringue, the mixture will eventually turn watery.

Make the Mango Gel

1. In a small saucepan, pour the mango puree over the agar; do not stir or heat. Set aside for 10 minutes or longer to allow the agar to hydrate.
2. Add sugar and lemon juice. Bring to a simmer, whisking frequently for a couple of minutes until sugar has dissolved. Make sure you whisk the bottom and the walls of the pot.
3. Pour the mixture into a shallow bowl and cool to room temperature. Refrigerate 20 to 30 minutes, or until the gel is very firm. Once firm. Cut the agar gel in small cubes and blend the gel cubes thoroughly using an immersion blender until smooth.
4. Pass the fluid gel through a fine sieve.

5. Store in a sealed container or squeeze bottle in the fridge until ready to use.

To Serve

1. Transfer the mousse to a piping bag. In a small dessert glass, serve the mango gel, add mousse, more mango gel and garnish with diced fruit of your choice, I recommend dragon fruit, mango, kiwi, and berries. Finish with piped vegan meringue, edible flowers and fresh mint leaves.

To Keep

1. Store the mousse in an airtight container for up to 3 days.

4. Mango Guyabano (Soursop) Smoothie
Total Time: 15 Minutes

Ingredients

- 1 cup soursop (ripe Guyabano, soursop flesh, removed)
- 3 cups mango (fresh and ripe, cubes)
- 1 cup ice cubes (or more)
- 1/2 cup milk (optional)
- sugar (or Honey, to taste, optional)

Direction

1. Place all ingredients in a blender and process until thick and smooth. Adjust the sweetness to your taste or you may not even need to add sugar if you have very sweet mangoes. Enjoy immediately!

5. Refreshing Soursop Juice
Total Time: 20 Minutes

Ingredients

- 1 soursop (medium)
- 2 limes (medium, use lemon if you can't find lime)
- 4 cups water
- sugar (to taste)

6. Red and White Soursop Shakes
Total Time: 8 Minutes

Ingredients

- ounces soursop
- 1 cup low fat plain yogurt
- 1/2 cup fat free milk
- 4 cups ice (divided)
- 6 strawberries (medium, rinsed, cored and quartered, about 1 cup)
- 1 teaspoon Goya Lemon Juice

Directions

1. Add nectar, yogurt, milk and 3 cups ice to blender. Blend until smooth and frothy, about 2 minutes; divide evenly among 4 glasses.
2. Quickly rinse out blender and add strawberries, lemon juice and 1 cup ice.. Blend until smooth and frothy, about 1 minute.
3. Immediately spoon strawberry puree evenly over top of each shake. Serve.

7. Soursop Coconut Smoothie
Total Time: 8 Minutes

Ingredients

- 1 cup soursop (fresh pulp or frozen)
- 1/3 cup coconut (chunks)
- 1 cup coconut milk (or coconut water)
- ice cubes

Directions

1. Place all the ingredients in a blender cup (no seeds if using fresh soursop!) and work it for about 1-2 minutes.
2. Serve with coconut shavings and chia seeds

8. Jamaican Soursop Drink
Total Time: 25 Minutes

Ingredients

- 1 soursop (ripe, Guanabana)
- 1 can sweetened condensed milk
- 1 teaspoon grated nutmeg
- 2 tablespoons fresh lime juice
- 1 tablespoon vanilla extract
- 5 cups water

Directions

1. Peel the soursop by hand; put flesh in a large mixing bowl and remove all the seeds
2. Put fruit into blender; add 3 cups of water and puree
3. Pour puree into in the mixing bowl and add 2 to 3 more cups of water. (If you prefer a smooth drink, use a strainer and the additional water to remove fruit fibers.)
4. Add sweetened condensed milk, nutmeg, lime juice and vanilla and stir to blend (if you don't

    have a large blender, like me, you can use a
    hand blender to do the final mixing

5. Serve chilled with or without ice cubes. Add a
   dash of nutmeg to each glass before serving.

9. Soursop Punch
Total Time: 60 Minutes

Ingredients

- 1 soursop (fruit medium sized)
- 1 1/2 pints cold water
- 1 strip lime peel
- 400 grams condensed milk (amount to suit taste or 2, 400 g cans condensed milk, amount to suit taste)

Directions

1. wash & peel soursop.
2. Mash in bowl with lime peel.
3. gradually stir in 1 pint water.
4. mix well & strain throuogh muslin cloth.
5. Add other 1/2 pint water , repeat process, making sure all flavour is out.
6. Add condensed milk to taste for sweetness.
7. Chill well before serving over Ice.

10. Soursop Drink
Total Time: 20 Minutes

Ingredients

- 1 soursop (medium)
- 6 cups water
- 3 cups soursop (pulping the, the other 3 cups to make up the drink)
- 1 tablespoon lime juice
- 1/4 teaspoon vanilla extract (/ essence)
- 2 Angostura bitters (splashes of)
- sugar (to taste, approximately 1 cup)
- 1 pinch salt

Directions

1. Peel soursop with your hand and remove and discard the spongy center.
2. Mash the flesh in a bowl with three cups of water to remove all the seeds.
3. Press this pulp through a sieve, resulting in a smooth puree.
4. Add the rest of the water to the puree

5. Add lime juice, sugar, salt, vanilla extract and bitters.

6. Taste and adjust the flavor as needed.

7. Chill and serve with ice.

Made in United States
Troutdale, OR
02/28/2024

18049705R00030